COLON PROCEDURE RECIPES

LOW FIBER—LOW RESIDUE MEALS

BY:

M.D. WELLS

Colon Procedure Recipes
Low Fiber—Low Residue Meals

Library of Congress Control Number: 2024902063

ISBN- 978-0-9706661-3-0

First edition 2024
Printed in the United States of America

Cover Image:Covenant Freelance Services via Canva.com
Cover Photo:©Africa-Images via Canva.com

Medical Disclaimer: I am not a health care practitioner. ALL
information in this book is purely for informational and educational
purposes. If you have any questions, please do your own research or
consult with your healthcare practitioner.

Publisher
Covenant Freelance Services
472 N. Ramos Lane
Green Valley, AZ 85614
USA

DEDICATION

ଚ୬

To All Physicians Aiding Our GI Health

This book is dedicated to the men and women who have dedicated their lives and professions to improving our gastrointestinal health.

Whether due to heredity, disease, diet, age, or our own propensity for bad behavior, they intervene to mitigate the consequences.

Their specialized training in the operation of our digestive organs has helped many of us to live longer, fuller lives. For this, we are exceedingly grateful.

CONTENTS

FOREWORD

After six days in the hospital following colon surgery, I couldn't even look at another bowl of lime jello or meat broth. I am so grateful for a caregiver who was willing to add variety to a very restrictive pre and post surgical diet. The meals suggested in this book made the process of recovery less odious and depressing. These tasty recipes made a bland diet much more enjoyable.

This is not a step-by-step gourmet cookbook. Through personal experience, Ms. Wells developed a specialized guide designed to aid meal planning in the interim to 'normal' eating. It will act as a quick, daily reference to simple meal ideas designed to meet the guidelines for colon recovery. It is easily organized into Breakfast, Lunch, Dinner and Snacks. It includes side-by-side sample meal choices as you transition between soft and low residue diets.

What can I say? Pudding is good but Peach Jello Mousse is even better. Raw carrots are not allowed but Carrot Soufflé is mouth watering. Chicken broth is boring but five choices of pureed soup is a welcome relief. Try everything!

I only hope this little book makes it to doctors' waiting rooms where it will benefit more patients like me.

Ed Brown
Delphi Electrical Engineer, Retired

PREFACE

Whether you are scheduled for a simple colonoscopy, or a surgical procedure, this book is for you.

When my husband was scheduled for a colon resection, I searched the internet for more information. I realized a special diet would be required, not only prior to the procedure, but for weeks following the procedure. I found only general information. I didn't find ideas for recipes to make the process easier and more enjoyable. That's when I decided to record our experience and the recipes we enjoyed.

Each procedure and each individual is different. Take things at your own pace. My husband had a robotic right hemicolectomy with approximately eight inches of colon removed. He was discharged from the hospital on the fifth post-op day, still unable to eat very much. On the eighth day following surgery my husband was able to eat one scrambled egg for breakfast, followed by a small amount of homemade chicken noodle soup for both lunch and dinner. Then it progressed from there.

Be encouraged. You will get back to 'normal' in time. This book will make the journey more enjoyable.

SPECIAL DIETS

Your physician will recommend a low residue diet prior to a colon procedure. This is similar to a low fiber diet but also limits a few other things, such as milk. This diet makes it easier for the prep to do its job in cleaning out the colon. Following intestinal surgery, it will also lessen irritation to the gastrointestinal tract and aid in healing.

It is usually recommended that you follow a low residue (low fiber) diet for five days prior to colonoscopy or colon surgery. A soft diet followed by a low residue diet will be recommended following colon surgery. It is also recommended that you eat smaller meals more frequently, like six times per day, every two to three hours.

Once your physician gives you the 'all clear,' you can slowly begin re-introducing fibrous foods. Use common sense. If a particular food makes you feel bad one or two hours later, stop eating it and try again in another week. Recovery can vary widely in each individual.

Remember, this isn't necessarily considered a healthy diet. It isn't meant for long term use because it lacks fiber and many nutrients.

Note: People with colostomy or ileostomy bags should consult a registered dietician.

Soft Diet: A good rule of thumb is, if you can't mash it with a fork, don't eat it.

Low Residue Diet: This refers to how much food is left in the colon after it is digested. The goal is fewer, smaller bowel movements daily. Avoid foods that are grainy, such as seeds, nuts, and raw vegetables high in fiber (peas, Brussels sprouts, broccoli). Avoid wholegrain breads or cereals such as oatmeal, buckwheat and popcorn. Avoid the skin and seeds of fruits and vegetables such as tomatoes, cucumbers, strawberries, pineapple, etc. No dried fruits such as prunes, raisins or figs.

Gas Producing Foods: Carbonated drinks, beans, dairy, and bread can produce gas which is more painful after surgery. Examples are corn, beans, lentils, peas, onions, garlic, broccoli, cauliflower, cabbage, sauerkraut, kale and tofu.

Fatty and greasy foods are also subject to producing abdominal pain and nausea.

Milk or dairy in moderation as this can trigger diarrhea and cramping. Cheese can cause constipation and therefore, bowel blockages. Use in moderation.

Chocolate can also be a potential trigger for gas, cramping and diarrhea. It contains a lot of sugar or sucrose and fat. Milk sugar also contains lactose, known to aggravate bowel symptoms.

Spicy foods and horseradish can irritate your digestive system and cause diarrhea or uncomfortable bloating. Cinnamon is a natural blood thinner and can cause post operative bleeding. Use nutmeg instead which is actually healthy for the digestive tract.

Sugar: Limit sugar intake after surgery. High sugar levels in the blood are known to inhibit the healing process. Also beware of artificial sweeteners which can cause an imbalance in the gut bacteria. This includes sorbitol, sucralose (Splenda), aspartame (Equal), and saccharin (Sweet'N Low).

Alcohol causes three problems. First, it hinders the body's ability to heal. Secondly it interferes with pain medications. Thirdly, it stimulates the intestines and causes more frequent bowel movements.

Omega-3: Fish Oil & Omega-3 fatty acids are often stopped prior to surgery to reduce the risk of bleeding. However, they can be resumed after your procedure. These aid in immune function and help to reduce inflammation.

Herbal Supplements: Your physician will advise you regarding certain supplements which interfere with blood clotting factors. Some have natural blood thinning properties and some interfere with other drugs being administered. Some of these include: aloe, cranberry, feverfew, garlic oil, ginger, ginkgo, turmeric, dong quail, evening primrose and ginseng.

Probiotics help restore gut health and can be helpful to your recovery.

Risk of Food Poisoning: While your colon is healing, it is best to avoid foods that carry any risk of food poisoning such as: non-pasteurized cheese, undercooked meats, sushi, fruits or vegetables not thoroughly washed.

Chew Food Thoroughly: Eat slowly, especially as you try to introduce new foods. If you chew to almost liquid consistency, it will be much easier for your colon to digest.

A healthy colon is able to absorb liquid. This process may be hindered during the healing process resulting in diarrhea and dehydration. Foods that are easy to digest help to reduce diarrhea. These include:
• ripe bananas
• soft cantaloupe or honeydew
• applesauce
• canned pears & peaches, no skin
• low sugar, low fiber cereal like puffed rice
• cream of rice or cream of wheat

- potatoes (white or sweet), no skin
- cooked beets, eggplant & mushrooms
- spinach
- canned green beans
- boiled white rice
- pasta
- tomato sauce (no seeds)
- creamy peanut butter
- mild cheese or cottage cheese
- white bread or toast
- pretzels (not whole grain)
- tapioca or smooth yogurt
- angel food cake
- canned or cooked fruits without seeds or skin
- ice cream, sherbet or frozen yogurt

Condiments allowed:
- margarine
- butter
- cream
- sour cream
- oils
- ketchup
- soy sauce
- mayonnaise
- mild salad dressings
- clear jelly
- honey
- syrup

Protein: Protein helps your body to heal and fight infection. Eat digestible proteins like eggs, lean meats, fish, poultry, cheese, yogurt, milk, nut butters, tofu, certain legumes such as chickpeas, lentils and kidney beans. Have a source of protein at each meal or snack. Limit dairy to two cups per day.

Drinks: Coffee and tea. Caffeine has been shown to enhance bowel recovery after surgery. Go easy, too much can trigger diarrhea and dehydration. Juices made without seeds or pulp. Strained vegetable juices. If you are not eating well, you need a source of salt and electrolytes like Gatorade®, Powerade® Ion4 or Pedialyte®.

Food Coloring: Red, purple and blue coloring can stain the walls of the colon. These stains can interfere with the procedure and look like blood or other abnormalities. Avoid drinks, jello, etc. with these colors.

Water: Drink 8-10 glasses of water per day.

As you transition to a regular diet, introduce fiber back into your diet gradually. The recommended amount is about five grams per week.

This cookbook is designed to give you cooking ideas and recipes for your journey back to colon health.

BREAKFAST

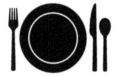

BREAKFAST

....

Peach Smoothie

1 cup white grape or apple juice

1 banana

1 small peach yogurt

1 cup frozen peach slices

• Place all ingredients in a blender and blend at high speed until smooth.

Scrambled Egg

1 large egg

1 teaspoon milk

salt & pepper

1 tablespoon shredded cheese (optional)

1 tablespoon butter

• Whisk egg, milk, seasonings & cheese together.
• Melt butter in a small skillet over medium heat. Pour egg mixture into pan and stir a little while cooking.

White Toast & Honey

• Toast a slice of bread
• Spread with pure honey
• Slice in long strips making it easier to eat

Avocado Toast

white toast

1 avocado

salt

- Cut avocado in half, remove the pit. Scoop the flesh into a bowl.
- Add a pinch of salt per avocado half. Mash with a fork. Spread onto toast and save the rest for later.

Pancakes and Waffles

all purpose baking mix

low sugar syrup

- Follow the recipe for pancakes or waffles on the box. Remember to go easy on syrup with sugar.

French Toast

2 large eggs

1/2 cup milk

2 teaspoons vanilla extract

pinch of nutmeg

pinch of salt

2 slices white bread, slightly stale

1 tablespoon butter and 1 tablespoon oil

- Whisk the eggs, milk, vanilla, nutmeg & salt in a bowl.
- Arrange bread in a shallow dish and pour the egg mixture on top. Let soak 10 minutes, turn over and soak 10 minutes.
- Heat the butter & oil in a skillet. Fry toast 2-3 minutes per side until golden. Serve with syrup or pureed fruit.

Deviled Eggs

6 hard-boiled eggs, peeled
1/4 cup mayonnaise or salad dressing
1 teaspoon mustard or dijon mustard
1/2 teaspoon white vinegar
1/4 teaspoon salt
2 teaspoons green onion, finely chopped
optional paprika

- Slice eggs in half. Gently scoop out yolks into a mixing bowl. Add all ingredients except paprika. Mix well.
- Re-fill sliced egg halves and sprinkle with paprika before serving.

Secret to Easy Peel Hard-Boiled Eggs

- Leave eggs cold in the refrigerator
- Bring water to boiling
- Carefully immerse cold eggs in boiling water. You can use tongs or a gravy ladle.
- Reduce to simmer. Simmer eggs 13 minutes.
- Just before eggs are finished, prepare an ice bath in a large bowl. Remove the eggs with tongs or ladle and immerse in ice bath. Let sit in ice bath 15 minutes.
- Gently rolls the egg back and forth along the counter with the palm of your hand. The peel will easily separate.

LUNCH

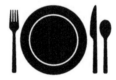

LUNCH

....

Beverages

Strained vegetable juice (like V8)

Gatorade® or Powerade® (avoid red & purple)

Pureed Soups Rich in Vitamins A, C & Zinc

Vitamins A, C, and Zinc help your body to repair tissue damage and fight infection.

Most pureed soups start with the "magic three" onion, celery and carrot. A chemical reaction occurs when these are sautéed together which greatly enhances flavor. However, in recipes for colon procedures, go very easy on the onion, or omit it.

In pureed soups, always stir the cream in by hand, at the end, after power blending, so as not to 'break' the cream. This is a term for causing the cream to separate.

Regular crackers can be served on a low residue diet. Cracked wheat or whole grain crackers are not allowed.

Vitamin A: carrot, sweet potato and spinach.

Vitamins A & C: potato, tomato and yellow squash

Zinc: chickpeas (garbanzo beans) and spinach

Creamy Potato Soup

2 pounds Russet potatoes, peeled, cubed
2 tablespoons salted butter
1/4 cup finely chopped onion
2 large carrots, peeled, finely chopped
2 celery stalks, finely chopped
1 box, low sodium, chicken broth
1 cup heavy cream
salt, pepper, Mrs. Dash original

- In a large pot, sauté onion, carrot & celery in butter until softened. Season with a little salt.
- Add potatoes and cover with chicken broth & water. Season with more salt, pepper, and Mrs. Dash.
- Bring to simmer. Cover and cook until vegetables are very tender, at least one hour.
- Puree completely with hand emulsion blender, or in small batches in a regular blender.
- Stir in heavy cream by hand and check seasoning. If you prefer thicker soup, dissolve some flour in the cream before adding to the pot or add instant potato flakes.

Creamy Yellow Squash Soup

- Use Creamy Potato Soup recipe above.
- Omit one pound potatoes and add 3 medium yellow squash, peeled and cubed.
- Thicken as above.

Creamy Sweet Potato Soup
- Use Creamy Potato Soup recipe (this section).
- Substitute 1 pound sweet potatoes (no skin).
- Thicken if necessary by adding some flour to the cream or add instant potato flakes.

Creamy Spinach Soup
- Use Creamy Potato Soup recipe (this section).
- Use 1 pound russet potatoes and add 1 pound spinach, thick stems trimmed.
- Thicken if necessary by adding some flour to the cream or add instant potato flakes.

Peanut Butter & Jelly Sandwich
- Creamy peanut butter only (no peanuts)
- Jelly only (no jam)
- Low fiber white bread, cut off the crust.

Chicken Salad Sandwich
- Canned chicken packed in water or shredded chicken
- Small amount of carrot & celery only if chopped ultra fine
- Mayonnaise or salad dressing to taste
- Pinch of salt
- Low fiber white bread, cut off the crust

<u>Modified Hummus — No Garlic</u>

1 can (15oz) chickpeas, drained, reserve 1/4 to 1/2 cup
chickpea liquid
1/3 cup tahini paste (sesame seed paste)
1/4 cup lemon juice (about 1 lemon, squeezed)
1 teaspoon sea salt
1 teaspoon garlic powder in lieu of fresh garlic
crackers, plain, low fiber, like saltine (limit 5 per day)

- Thoroughly stir tahini before measuring to incorporate oil that naturally settles to the top.
- In a high powered food processor, blend the drained chickpeas to a creamy consistency. Pause periodically to scrape the sides, center and bottom of bowl to ensure all chickpeas are processed. If mixture appears too thick, add some reserved chickpea liquid.
- Add Tahini paste and blend to combine.
- Add lemon juice and sea salt. Stop to scrape sides and then process until very creamy.
- Before serving, drizzle with a little olive oil and sprinkle with paprika, if desired.
- Serve with saltine crackers or other mild cracker.

Sloppy Joes

1 pound hamburger

1/8 cup sugar

1 teaspoon vinegar

1/2 teaspoon prepared mustard

1/2 cup ketchup

1/4 cup BBQ sauce

1/2 teaspoon salt

- Brown hamburger and drain.
- Add remaining ingredients.
- Simmer 1/2 hour. Serve on plain white hamburger buns.

DINNER

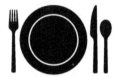

DINNER

··

Simple, Plain Pasta

- Use plain white pasta, spaghetti, or angel hair. Do <u>not</u> use whole grain pasta.
- Top with butter and salt
- Or top with small amount of Alfredo sauce (this section)
- Or top with small amount of Secret Sauce (this section)

Pasta with Modified Pesto

2 cups chopped fresh basil, stems removed

1/4 cup grated parmesan cheese

2 tablespoons lemon juice

1/8 cup extra virgin olive oil (use the good stuff)

1/4 teaspoon salt

Note that pine nuts & fresh garlic have been omitted

- Pulse in food processor until creamy.
- Serve over fine spaghetti noodles or angel hair pasta.

Macaroni and Cheese

- Use a good brand of boxed macaroni & cheese.
- I personally think home made is a lot of work.
- If making your favorite home-made mac & cheese, go easy on the cheese as it can cause constipation.

Easy Fettuccine Alfredo

• Boiled fettuccine noodles and top with a jar of warmed Alfredo sauce (homemade or jar).

Homemade Alfredo Sauce

2 tablespoons olive oil
1 tablespoon flour
1-1/2 cups milk
1 cup freshly grated parmesan cheese
2 tablespoons cream cheese
1/2 teaspoon salt
1 teaspoon garlic powder (omit fresh garlic)
pepper to taste

• Heat olive oil in medium saucepan over medium heat.
• Stir in flour. Gradually add milk, whisking continuously until mixture thickens, about 6 minutes.
• Add parmesan cheese, cream cheese and seasonings, whisking until cheese melts.
• Serve on fettuccine noodles.

Chicken Fettuccine Alfredo

chicken breast, cooked, cut in strips or chunks
fettuccine noodles, boiled, drained
jar of Alfredo sauce or homemade (above)
1/4 cup freshly grated parmesan cheese

• Combine the pasta, chicken and sauce. Sprinkle with extra parmesan cheese before serving.

Middle Eastern White Rice

2 tablespoons butter

1 cup extra fine egg noodles

1 cup white rice (Basmati rice preferred)

2 cups chicken broth

1 teaspoon salt

- Melt butter in saucepan. Add fine egg noodles. Stir until browned in color. Watch closely as they will burn quickly.
- Add rice and chicken broth. Cover and simmer until liquid is absorbed, about 20 minutes.

Easy Mashed Potatoes

2 pounds Russet or Idaho potatoes

1/4 cup salted real butter (no substitutes)

1/4 cup milk, room temperature

1/4 cup cream or Greek yogurt, room temperature

salt & pepper to taste

- Peel and cube potatoes. Place in saucepan and cover with cold water. Bring to a boil and cook until tender 15-20 minutes. Drain.
- Add butter, milk, cream, salt and pepper.
- Mash with hand masher or potato ricer. If using electric mixer, be careful not to over mix which causes a gummy texture.

Potato Puff For Two

2 baking potatoes, peeled and cubed
1/2 cup small curd cottage cheese
1 egg
1/2 cup dairy sour cream
1/8 cup green onion, very small dice
2 tablespoons butter, softened
1/2 teaspoon salt
dash pepper (optional)

- Preheat oven to 325°.
- Cook potatoes in boiling salted water for 20 minutes or until very tender. Drain and mash.
- Butter two single-serving casserole dishes.
- In a large bowl, beat cottage cheese and eggs at high speed until almost smooth.
- At low speed, beat in sour cream, green onions, softened butter, salt and pepper.
- Add potatoes and beat until well blended.
- Transfer to baking dishes. Drizzle top with a little more melted butter. Bake 40-50 minutes or until heated in center and top is lightly browned.

Carrot Soufflés

1 pounds carrots, peeled & cut in pieces
1/2 pound yams (sweet potatoes), cut in pieces
3/4 cup butter
3 large eggs
1/4 cup all-purpose flour
1/2 tablespoon baking powder
1-1/2 cups sugar
1/2 tablespoon vanilla
powdered sugar (optional)

- Cook carrots and sweet potatoes in boiling water for 15-20 minutes, until tender. Drain.
- In food processor with knife blade, add carrots, yams, and all remaining ingredients, except powdered sugar. Process until smooth, stopping once to scrape sides.
- Spoon into a lightly greased 1-1/2 quart soufflé or baking dish. Sprinkle with powdered sugar if desired.
- Bake 350º for 1 hour or until set and lightly browned.

Green Bean Casserole

1 can cream of mushroom soup
1/2 cup milk
4 cups canned french-style green beans, drained
1-1/3 cups french-fried onions

- Heat oven to 350º. Prepare 1-1/2 quart casserole dish.
- Mix soup, milk, beans and 2/3 cup french-fried onions.
- Bake 25 minutes. Stir. Top with remaining french-fried onions and bake 5 minutes more.

Spinach Casserole

3 tablespoons unsalted butter
1/4 cup finely chopped green onion
1-1/4 cups heavy cream
2 (10oz) packages frozen chopped spinach
1/2 teaspoon salt
1/2 cup grated parmesan cheese, divided
1/4 cup sour cream
2 tablespoons Panko bread crumbs

* Preheat oven to 400º.
* Spray or grease a 1-1/2 to 2 quart casserole.
* Drain spinach and squeeze dry.
* Melt butter in saucepan over medium heat. Add green onion to soften. Add cream and bring to a simmer. Stir occasionally until slightly thickened, about 5 minutes. Mix in the spinach, salt and 1/4 cup parmesan cheese. Add cream cheese and stir until melted.
* Transfer to prepared baking dish. Sprinkle with bread crumbs and remaining 1/4 cup parmesan cheese.
* Bake until bubbling and light golden brown, about 15 minutes.

Chicken Breast & Penne in Secret Sauce

Marinade Chicken

2 boneless, skinless chicken breast halves

1/2 tablespoon olive oil

1/2 tablespoon lemon pepper rub

- Cut chicken breasts in half crosswise and pound thin.
- Rub oil on both sides. Sprinkle with lemon pepper.
- Cover with plastic wrap. Rest until sauce is ready.

Secret Sauce

2 tablespoons butter	2 tablespoons flour
1 cup chicken stock	1/2 teaspoon salt
1/2 teaspoon Mrs. Dash	1/2 cup sour cream
1-1/2 tablespoons lemon juice	1/2 cup mayonnaise

1/2 cup fresh parmesan cheese, grated

- Melt butter in skillet, add flour and stir until bubbly.
- Add stock, spices & lemon juice. Add all remaining ingredients. Heat through. Cover and set aside.

Chicken & Penne

2 cups Penne pasta

1/4 cup finely chopped onion

- Boil water and cook pasta.
- Heat oil in skillet. Dust chicken with flour & fry in hot oil until done (about 4 min. per side). Remove to plate.
- Add onion to skillet and cook 1 minute. Add 1/2 the sauce and heat until bubbly. Return chicken to pan. Cover and simmer 2 minutes more.
- Serve pasta with remaining secret sauce.

Oven Baked Chicken Fingers

2 boneless, skinless chicken breasts
2/3 cup baking mix, like Bisquick
1/2 cup grated parmesan cheese
1/2 teaspoon garlic salt
1/2 teaspoon paprika
1 egg, whisked
3 tablespoons butter, melted

- Preheat oven to 450º. Cut chicken breasts into 1/2 inch strips across the grain.
- Combine baking mix, parmesan, salt & paprika in a bag. Dip chicken strips in egg wash, then shake in bag.
- Place in well-greased pan. Drizzle with melted butter.
- Bake for 12-14 min. Turn pieces over half way through.

Sour Cream Meatloaf

1 lb. hamburger	1/2 cup sour cream
1/2 tsp. salt	1 egg
1/8 tsp. pepper	1 tsp. mustard
1/8 cup sugar	1 Tbsp. parsley
1 Tbsp. Worcestershire	1/2 cup ketchup

1/2 cup Townhouse crackers, crushed (about 12)
1/4 cup old fashioned rolled oats

- Preheat oven to 375º.
- Spray a loaf pan with non-stick spray.
- Mix all ingredients well. Shape into a loaf in the pan.
- Top with additional 1/2 cup of ketchup if desired.
- Bake 50 minutes. Cool 5-10 minutes before serving.

Honey Mustard Turkey Meatballs

1 pound ground turkey

1 egg

3/4 cup butter flavored crackers, crushed

6 tablespoons Dijon mustard, divided

1/2 teaspoon ground ginger

1/2 cup shredded mozzarella cheese

1-1/4 cups unsweetened, strained, pineapple juice

2 tablespoons honey

1 tablespoon cornstarch

1/4 teaspoon onion powder

- In a bowl, combine turkey, egg, crackers, 3 Tbsp. mustard, ginger and cheese. Form into 30 (1") balls.
- Place in greased 13 X 9 pan & bake uncovered at 350° for 20-25 minutes or until juices run clear.
- In a saucepan, combine pineapple juice, honey, cornstarch and onion powder. Bring to boil, stirring constantly. Cook & stir 2 minutes more. Reduce heat.
- Stir in remaining 3 tablespoons mustard until smooth.
- Brush meatballs with about 1/4 cup of sauce and return to the oven for ten minutes.
- Serve with remaining sauce for dipping.

Pressure-Cooked Beef or Pork

• Use a pressure cooker for roasts of beef or pork. This makes them very tender and more digestible.
• If using onion, carrot, or celery for flavor, remove and discard before serving.

Ritz Fish

1 pound fish (sole, perch, scrod, or other mild fish)
4 tablespoons unsalted butter
2/3 cup crushed Ritz crackers
1/4 cup grated parmesan cheese
1/2 teaspoon dried basil
1/2 teaspoon dried oregano
1/4 teaspoon garlic powder

• Melt butter in a 9 X 13 baking pan.
• Combine all ingredients, except fish, in a bag.
• Dip the fish around the melted butter, then into the crumb mixture. Return to baking dish.
• Bake uncovered 350º for 20-25 minutes.

DESSERTS & SNACKS

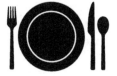

DESSERTS & SNACKS

....

Sherbet (avoid red, blue & purple)

Popsicles (avoid red, blue & purple)

Jello (avoid red, blue & purple)

Pudding

Custard

Cottage Cheese

Applesauce (no cinnamon)

Canned fruits such as peaches, pears or mandarin oranges (no pineapple, no seeds or skins)

Bananas

Soft Melons (no watermelon which can aggravate gas, bloating and loose stools)

Avocado

Whipped Cottage Cheese
1 cup cottage cheese
2 teaspoons honey
1 teaspoon vanilla

- Whip in food processor or blender.
- Chill in refrigerator

Peach Jello Mousse

1 package peach Jello (4 serving size)
1/2 cup boiling water
1 cup canned peaches, drained
1/2 cup cream cheese, softened, cubed
1/2 cup cold water
1/4 teaspoon vanilla extract
1 cup Cool Whip

- Add Jello package to a medium bowl. Pour in boiling water and stir until completely dissolved.
- Pour Jello mixture into a blender or food processor. Add peaches, cream cheese, vanilla extract and cold water. Blend until smooth, about one minute.
- Pour into a large mixing bowl. Whisk in the Cool Whip by hand until completely blended. Distribute into four dessert dishes. Refrigerate until set, about 2 hours.

Homemade Peanut Butter Pudding

1/3 cup sugar
1/4 teaspoon salt
1/2 cup half and half cream
1/2 cup creamy peanut butter

4-1/2 tsp. cornstarch
1-1/2 cups milk
1 tsp. vanilla extract

- In a saucepan, combine sugar, cornstarch, and salt.
- Gradually stir in milk and cream; bring to a boil over medium heat. Cook and stir for 2 minutes.
- Remove from heat; stir in peanut butter and vanilla until smooth. Pour into serving dishes and refrigerate.

Homemade Banana Pudding
(For Southern Banana Pudding or Banana Cream Pie)

2 large bananas
1/2 cup sugar
1/3 cup all-purpose flour
1/4 teaspoon salt
2 cups milk
3 egg yolks, slightly beaten
2 tablespoons unsalted butter
1 teaspoon vanilla
vanilla wafers or baked 9" pie crust
Cool Whip topping

- In a saucepan, combine sugar, flour and salt. Gradually stir in the milk. Cook and stir over medium heat until mixture boils and thickens. Cook 2 minutes more.
- Remove from heat. Stir a small amount of hot liquid into the egg yolks to temper them (otherwise they will cook). Then stir the yolks into the hot mixture and cook 2 more minutes, stirring constantly.
- Remove from heat. Add butter and vanilla.

For Southern Banana Pudding: Line bottom and sides of an individual serving dish with vanilla wafers. Top with sliced banana. Top with pudding. Makes 4 servings

For Pie: Line bottom and sides of a cooled pastry shell with sliced bananas. Pour pudding over top of bananas. Refrigerate about a half hour. Top with Cool Whip and serve.

Peanut Butter and Jelly Mini Muffins

2 eggs

1/2 cup plain or vanilla yogurt

3 tablespoons creamy peanut butter

2 tablespoons vegetable oil or olive oil

1 cup flour

1/3 cup firmly packed brown sugar

1 teaspoon baking powder

1/2 teaspoon baking soda

1/4 teaspoon salt

3 tablespoon favorite jelly (no jam)

- In a large mixing bowl, combine eggs, yogurt, peanut butter and oil on low speed until smooth.
- In separate mixing bowl, whisk together flour, sugar, baking powder, soda and salt.
- Stir dry ingredients into wet ingredients just until moistened.
- Fill greased miniature muffin cups half full. Top each with 1/4 teaspoon jelly. Add remaining batter on top of each.
- Bake 400° for 10 to 12 minutes, until golden brown.
- Cool 5 minutes before removing.
- Note: Regular size muffins use 3/4 teaspoon jelly and bake 12-14 minutes.

Banana Bread

1/2 cup sugar

1/2 cup oil

2 eggs

1-1/4 cups flour

1/2 teaspoon baking powder

1/2 teaspoon baking soda

1/2 teaspoon salt

NO cinnamon (it can cause bleeding)

1 teaspoon vanilla

1 cup mashed ripe banana

- Preheat oven to 350°.
- In a large bowl, mix together sugar, oil and eggs.
- In a separate bowl, mix dry ingredients together.
- Add dry ingredients to wet ingredients. Mix well.
- Add vanilla and mashed banana. Place into a greased medium sized loaf pan.
- Bake for 30-40 minutes. Toothpick inserted in center should come out clean.

<u>Applesauce Cake</u>

1 egg

1/3 cup vegetable oil or olive oil

1/2 cup plain Greek yogurt

1/2 cup unsweetened applesauce (no cinnamon)

1 teaspoon vanilla extract

1-1/4 cups all-purpose flour

2/3 cup firmly packed brown sugar

NO cinnamon (it can cause bleeding)

1/2 teaspoon nutmeg (good for digestion)

3/4 teaspoon baking powder

3/4 teaspoon baking soda

1/4 teaspoon salt

Powdered sugar for dusting (optional)

- Preheat oven to 350°. Grease an 8 inch square pan.
- In a large bowl, mix together egg, oil, yogurt, applesauce and vanilla.
- In a separate bowl, whisk together the flour, brown sugar, baking powder, baking soda and salt.
- Add the dry ingredients to the wet ingredients and blend thoroughly.
- Pour into prepared pan and smooth the top.
- Bake 25-30 minutes until toothpick inserted in center comes out clean.
- Dust with powdered sugar while still warm.
- Cool 1 hour and cut into squares.

Moist Banana Cake

9 X 13 pan	8 X 8 pan
4 bananas, mashed	2 bananas, mashed
2 tsp. lemon juice	1 tsp. lemon juice
3 cups all purpose flour	1-1/2 cups flour
1-1/2 tsp. baking soda	3/4 tsp. baking soda
1/4 tsp. salt	1/8 tsp. salt
3/4 cup butter, softened	6 Tbsp. butter, softened
1/2 cup sugar	1/4 cup sugar
3 large eggs	2 small eggs
2 tsp. vanilla extract	1 tsp. vanilla extract
1-1/2 cups buttermilk	3/4 cup buttermilk
Powdered sugar for dusting	(Same)

Note: Buttermilk substitute: 1 teaspoon vinegar or lemon juice added to 1 cup milk. Let stand 5 minutes.

- Preheat oven to 275°. Grease pan.
- Mash bananas with lemon juice, set aside.
- In separate bowl, whisk together flour, soda and salt.
- In large bowl, with electric mixer, cream butter and sugar together until light and fluffy, about 3 minutes.
- Add eggs to sugar mixture, one at a time, then vanilla.
- Add half of the flour mixture and all of the buttermilk, then add remainder of flour.
- Stir in mashed bananas.
- Pour into prepared baking pan. Bake 55-60 minutes.
- Dust with powdered sugar immediately.
- Secret: For very moist cake, immediately place pan in freezer for 45 minutes.

Lemon Angel Food Cake

1 box Angel Food cake mix (16 oz. "add water only" variety)
1 can (21 oz.) lemon pie filling

• Preheat oven to 350°
• Grease or spray a 9 X 13 pan.
• In large bowl, add the cake mix and entire can of lemon pie filling (no water is added). Using a wire whip, mix gently until moistened, then beat until fluffy and fully combined.
• Pour into prepared pan and bake 30 minutes. Top will be fluffy and cracked but settles after cooling.
• Cool 15 minutes. Serve with optional whipped cream.

Note: This would also work with other pie fillings but avoid red or purple fruits and no fruit with seeds or skin.

Angel Food Cake with Peach Topping

1 box Angel Food cake mix
1 can of peach pie filling

• Make cake according to box directions.
• Puree the can of peach pie filling until smooth and serve as topping.

Peach Cream Pie

2 large eggs, slightly beaten

1/3 cup flour

1/2 cup sugar

Pinch of salt

1 cup heavy whipping cream

1 teaspoon vanilla extract

3 cups peaches, skin removed, thinly sliced

1 unbaked pie shell

- Preheat oven to 375º.
- Arrange peaches in the pie crust.
- In a small bowl, whisk eggs, sugar, flour and salt.
- Whisk in cream and vanilla. Pour over peaches.
- Bake 40-50 minutes. Cover edge of crust with foil when browned to prevent over browning.
- Chill 20 minutes before serving. Refrigerate leftovers.

Peanut Butter No Bake Cookies

1/4 cup brown sugar	1/4 cup white sugar
1/2 cup light corn syrup	3/4 cup peanut butter
1 teaspoon vanilla	2 cups Rice Krispies

- Combine all ingredients.
- Drop by teaspoonfuls onto waxed paper until set.
- Don't eat the whole batch. Be moderate with sugar.

Peanut Butter Rice Krispies Treats

4 tablespoons unsalted butter

1/4 teaspoon vanilla

1/4 teaspoon salt

2/3 cup creamy peanut butter

1 (10oz) package mini marshmallows

6 cups Rice Krispies or rice cereal

- Separate marshmallows into 5 cups and 2 cups.
- Melt butter over low heat. Add salt, vanilla and peanut butter until melted. Stir in 5 cups marshmallows until smooth and creamy.
- Add rice cereal and last 2 cups of marshmallows until combined. This will leave a few bits of undissolved marshmallows visible in the mix.
- Press into a 9 X 13 greased pan. A piece of waxed paper is good for pressing.
- Cool to room temperature. Slice and serve.

Success Keys: Use low heat. Do not over stir. Do not compact too hard.

SAMPLE
CHOICES

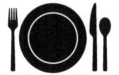

SAMPLE CHOICES

....

BREAKFAST
SOFT DIET

Coffee or Juice
Smoothie
Banana
Cream of Wheat Cereal
Cream of Rice Cereal
Scrambled egg with mild cheese

MID MORNING SNACK
SOFT DIET

Electrolyte Drink
Ensure®
6 ounces Apple Juice
Plain Jello (no red, blue or purple)
Yogurt
Whipped Cottage Cheese
Applesauce (no cinnamon)

SAMPLE CHOICES

....

BREAKFAST
LOW RESIDUE DIET

Anything on Soft Diet Menu—Plus:
White Toast and Honey or Jelly (no jam)
Avocado Toast
Pancake
Waffle
French Toast
Rice Cereal
Hard-boiled Egg
Deviled Egg

MID MORNING SNACK
LOW RESIDUE DIET

Anything on Soft Diet Menu—Plus:
White Toast with Honey or Jelly (no jam)
Cottage Cheese
Soft Melon (no watermelon)
Vanilla Wafers
Rice Krispies Treat

SAMPLE CHOICES

....

LUNCH
SOFT DIET

6 ounces White Grape Juice
Smoothie
Banana
Cantaloupe or Honey Dew Melon
Cottage Cheese
Pureed Soups (potato, squash, spinach)
Mashed Potatoes

MID AFTERNOON SNACK
LOW RESIDUE DIET

Anything on Mid-Morning Snacks—Plus:
Sherbet (no red, blue or purple)
Popsicle (no red, blue or purple)
Pudding
Custard

SAMPLE CHOICES

LUNCH
LOW RESIDUE DIET

Anything on Soft Diet Menu—Plus:
Vegetable Juice, like V8®
Peanut Butter & Jelly (on soft white bread)
Cooked White Rice
Chicken Noodle Soup
Chicken or Tuna Salad (on crackers or soft white bread)
Baked Potato, no skin (with butter & sour cream)
Sloppy Joe (on soft white bun)
Hamburger (ketchup or mayo on soft white, seedless bun)

MID AFTERNOON SNACK
LOW RESIDUE DIET

Anything on Mid-Morning Snacks—Plus:
3 Mini Muffins
Avocado
Hummus on Saltines
Vanilla Wafers
1 Peanut Butter No-Bake Cookie

SAMPLE CHOICES

....

DINNER
SOFT DIET

Anything on Lunch Menu—Plus:
6 ounces strained vegetable juice (like V8®)
Potato Puff (omit green onion)
Carrot Soufflé

SAMPLE CHOICES

DINNER
LOW RESIDUE DIET

Anything on Lunch Menu

Anything on Soft Diet Dinner Menu—Plus:

Macaroni & Cheese

Middle Eastern White Rice

Potato Puff

Pasta with Butter, Alfredo, Secret Sauce or Pesto

White Dinner Roll

Bread Stick

Green Bean Casserole

Spinach Casserole

Chicken Fettuccine Alfredo

Chicken Breast with Penne & Secret Sauce

Chicken Fingers

Meatloaf or Meatballs

Ritz Fish or Broiled Fish

Pressure-cooked Beef or Pork

SAMPLE CHOICES

....

EVENING SNACK
SOFT DIET

Anything on previous soft snack menus—Plus:
Peach Jello Mousse
Peanut Butter Pudding
Banana Pudding
Lemon Pudding
Angel Food Cake
Marshmallows

SAMPLE CHOICES

....

EVENING SNACK
LOW RESIDUE DIET

Anything on all previous snack menus—Plus:
Canned Fruits without seeds or skins (no pineapple)
Banana Bread
Banana Cream Pie
Peach Cream Pie
Applesauce Cake
Banana Cake

How to Order

....

Colon Procedure Recipes
Low Fiber—Low Residue Meals

Available on Amazon.com

Reviews on Amazon are always appreciated.

If you have suggestions for how to improve revised editions of this book, please feel free to email the author at M.D.Wells.USA@gmail.com

FREE OFFER

Join the email list for future offers and receive a free PDF flyer "Secrets To Successful Dry Pasta."

Email M.D.Wells.USA@gmail.com. Put "Pasta Secrets" in the Subject line and in the body, tell us where you found this book.

Printed in Great Britain
by Amazon

42008888R00036